The Patient's Guide to Pain Management

What You Need to Know to Navigate Through the Stigma to Get the Care that You Need

By

Harvey Jenkins MD PhD

Introduction

Why be a victim when you don't have to be?
Understanding how to navigate the complex maze
of pain-management care is difficult for people
who suffer from pain, particularly in the unfriendly,
sometimes hostile and increasingly repressive and
stigmatized environment surrounding pain
management today. It further victimizes people
who are already victims of their pain. This guide
for patients with pain simplifies this process,
allowing you to get the access you need to the right
medical professionals, to know what to expect from
them and to help you avoid and overcome the
common pitfalls that can sabotage your care. It is
written in a 'non-clinical' language that anyone can
understand. Everyone with pain, the people who
love them and the providers who care for them,
should read this book so that they will not remain a
victim of their pain.

Table of Contents

Chapter 1

Why You Need This Book

Statistically speaking you or someone you know is a victim of pain. It is estimated that 100 Million people in America are also victims, and suffer from some type of chronic pain, according to the Institute of Medicine. This translates into more than 600 billion dollars annually in medical costs and lost productivity. The sheer numbers of people with pain is even more than the number of people who suffer from cancer, heart-disease and diabetes combined. With these large numbers, you would think accessing care for pain would be simple. Instead, there are many obstacles and challenges to finding treatment for pain. These unfortunate challenges exist for several reasons: the lack of fundamental understanding and inability to access care by people who suffer from pain and the social stigma and other barriers which deter people with legitimate pain from accessing care. There is also a shortage of professionals who treat people with pain and a hesitation by other providers who could treat people with pain, due to repressive intrusion by regulations affecting pain treatment. This intrusion serves to "criminalize" patients who have pain and the prescribers who need to treat them. There is also an increasingly recognized inability of the policy-makers we elect to create and champion the kinds of legislation and policy measures that protect access to safe treatment, rather than misguided attempts of law which makes it harder to access.

At its root, the cause of these challenges lies in one basic fact: Too often, pain medication prescribed for treatment of pain is wrongfully equated with drug abuse, drug-selling, addiction, drug overdose, and self-destructive and anti-social behavior. What even reasonably well-educated people with good intentions who happen to believe these things don't always realize is that pain-management is none of these things. Yet, patients who suffer from pain are are often ostracized by their families and communities and treated as if they are addicts, abusers or criminals. This leads of lot of people to suffer in silence and avoid treatment. The silent suffering may lead to clinical depression and its consequences. The stresses that people will pain can have a direct impact on heart function, blood pressure, immunity as well as many other aspects of health. It can also lead to acts of desperation. It can lead to criminality. It can kill you.

What is needed to fix these problems is a consistent effort in educating people about the nature of pain, the importance of treatment, and the misguided social and legal barriers that prevent access to pain-management. Doing so, will not only alleviate suffering, improve the quality of lives, but actually save lives lost to street-drug overdoses and suicide, options that are taken when desperate attempts to legitimate and legal access to treatment is obstructed or denied.

By reading this book, you are probably one of pain's victims, directly or indirectly. You may be someone realizing that you need treatment but don't know where to start and what to do. You may be a family member or friend wanting to help a loved one in need. Maybe you are someone who wants to be a part of the policy change in your community to make things better, and you want a feel for the complexity of the issues regarding pain-management. Maybe you are health-care provider who wants to develop his or her reasonable expectations for your patients. If you fall in to any of these groups of people, this book will help you. And congratulations, because if you are one of these people, you are not just becoming 'part of the solution', you are the solution.

Chapter 2

Knowing your Pain and Communicating it Effectively

A. Knowing What Pain is

1. What is Pain?

Unfortunately, most of us know what Pain is. We don't need to grab the dictionary in order to formulate our own definition. On the other hand, to define our pain specifically, such that we can easily communicate to a family member or health-care professional may be challenging. The goal of this section is to provide you with the tools to define the pain you have, in the most accurate and specific terms possible, and to be able to communicate it to your doctor or health-care provider

If we look to our dictionary, Pain is defined as "physical suffering or discomfort caused by illness or injury". The pain is perceived or sensed by the part of the nervous system called the Peripheral nervous system and transmitted via other nerves in the central nervous system (spinal cord and brain), so that it may be modulated and interpreted by specialized regions of the brain. The processing of this information by the brain is what gives us the sensation of pain as well as the emotions that are associated with a painful episode or pain that does not go away. This definition of pain is adequate, but probably not helpful enough for most purposes. When you suffer from pain, and that suffering requires you to see a doctor, the definition seems to be limited. Understanding the limitation will allow you to not only define your pain better and communicate it in terms your doctor will understand.

2. What is Pain-management?

Pain Management is a branch of medicine which has as its goal to relieve pain, ease the suffering, and improve the quality of life with people who live with pain. Although the treatment of pain is not a new discipline, the field of pain management is in many ways still in its infancy. There are many areas of this field which lack consistency and standards like the more established subspecialties of medicine. Your provider, like many pain-management doctors, may have experience in treating pain from their basic medical and residency training with no certification. Your provider may have certification by the **American Board of Pain Medicine**, which requires no additional graduate medical training or by the **American Board of Anesthesiology, Physical Medicine and Rehabilitation(PMR, Physiatry)** and their Osteopathic Medicine equivalents, which is recognized by the **American Board if Medical Specialties** and does involve graduate medical training beyond their residency training. Because of the relative youth in this field, practitioners with or without specialized training, can participate harmoniously and very effectively in the grand scheme of pain treatment.

Although the Societies for Providers who treat pain do offer recommendations and guidelines for standards of care, too often, the practice of pain management is being increasingly regulated and, to some degree, forcibly limited by State and Regulatory Agencies such as **State Medical Boards** (which license physicians in your state), **State Bureaus for Narcotics, Controlled-Substances & Drugs that are classified as Dangerous, Law-Enforcement Agencies**, and, federally, by the **Drug Enforcement Agencies**

(DEA) and **Food & Drug Administration (FDA)**. Insurance companies may add to this regulatory force directly, by limiting which medications, some of which are expensive, that they will agree to authorize and cover. Likewise, medication availability, which had been previous unheard of with pain medications in past years, has tended to occur more regularly as shifts in laws and changes in the classification of certain pain medications becomes more regular. Pharmaceutical companies and manufacturers cannot keep up with demand of certain medications because of these changes. Pharmacies, both 'large-chain' and "Mom & Pop" smaller pharmacies may have their supplies of pain medications limited by their suppliers, or do so deliberately, to evade scrutiny by agencies which track their dispensing patterns. With the large number of regulatory forces controlling these medications, it is no surprise that policies can vary by location and be in direct conflict with each other.

Pain Management in its most basic form is your health-care provider or a physician who specializes in this discipline to whom you are referred. In the broadest sense, pain-management can take an interdisciplinary approach to pain treatment involving a variety of clinicians with different areas of an expertise. For example there may not only be your **pain management doctor** who is involved , but also **mid-level practitioners, nurses and assistants, Physical therapists, Occupational Therapists, Psychologists, Psychiatrists, Physiatrists, Neurologists, Internal Medicine Specialists, Interventional Pain specialists, Surgeons and Social Workers.** In some areas, chiropractors, acupuncturists, dietitians and holistic medicine specialists are available, particular when the patients indicate this type of treatment as their preference.

B.   Communicating your Pain Effectively to your Health-Care Provider

Now that you have the basic definitions in hand and an introduction to the scope of issues surrounding pain-management, it is appropriate to begin the process of interacting within that field. When you access treatment opportunity and you want the best possible, the first thing that needs to understood is how to communicate you pain. People who have pain communicate their pain experience all the time to spouses and partners and to their entire social network. That type of communication is appropriate in that context. However, when communicating you pain to a health-care provide, you must be more specific. These *descriptors* are the ones you will need to specify your pain to your provider so they can arrive at the correct diagnosis of your problem and offer you the most effective treatment plan.

1. **Location**

This is perhaps the easiest way to specify your pain. But, this is certainly not for everyone or all types of pain in the body. Usually the pain is specified by the **anatomical location.** The anatomical locations that are the most helpful are probably obvious to you; like the head, jaw, neck, back, chest, abdomen, pelvis, groin, arms, legs hands and feet. For example, most adults over 40 years old know what 'back pain' feels like, because it is perceived in the back. Many will also be what 'shoulder pain' is like, because it is perceived in the shoulder. Similarly, most people know what a headache feels like, but may have difficulty in pointing out what part of the head it is coming from. Migraine headache pain sometimes falls in to this category, although typically it is experienced on one side of the head only. Sinus pain and neck pain may also be perceived as headaches, although t he origins of this pain is different than the origin of the classic type of headache. Even more strange are the few patients I have encountered who have no concept of what a headache is like, because they have never actually had one.

A special type of pain called Phantom pain is the pain perceived in a limb or body part that has been amputated, is even harder to describe specifically.

Once you establish the location, it is necessary to clarify whether the pain is **focal**, or limited to one region or is **non-focal**. Not all pain is focal or limited to a specific area. Some pain types actually **travel** or **radiate** to other locations of the body. Some types of neck pain radiate down one or both arms. The principle behind radiating pain in the neck has to do with the route the nerve and its branches take down the arm or arms when the a nerve is being "pinched" by a bulging disk in the neck. When the term "sciatica" is used, it describes pain that may originate with a focal problem in back, but is *referred* to the buttock and down the back of the thigh and leg to varying degrees.

Pain is often **referred** to other places on the body, which mean that even though the pain originates in one location, it is perceived in another location. Back pain is sometimes referred to the notch you can feel on each side of the back of the pelvis called the Sacroiliac Joint region.

Beyond the regional anatomy, and the radiation or referral pattern, it is important to further define the location for some types of pain.

For example, the term "Back Pain" is less specific than "Low Back pain" or "Lumbar Pain", and is the pain involving the part of spine beneath the last rib and ends at the pelvis. This area is call the Lumbar spine. The part of the spine bearing ribs, which is occasionally but not frequently associated with pain is called the Thoracic Spine.

The Abdomen is a region that when pain is experienced is best subdivided into 4 quadrants: Right And Left Upper Quadrants, and Right and Left Lower Quadrants. The presence of pain in thee areas can help identify the source. For example pain in the "Right Upper Quadrant" may be due to a gallbladder problem, particularly if the pain can be intensified with deep pressure in this area.

Although less important, some clinicians find it easy to assess pain in the lower and upper extremities with names that may be different than the ones you use in conversation. For example, the upper extremity consists of the shoulder, the arm, the elbow joint, forearm, hand and fingers. Any of these locations can be painful, but saying "my 'arm' hurts", when you really mean "my forearm hurts" is not proper. Similarly the lower extremity is subdivided in to the hip, thigh, knee joint, leg, foot and toes. To say "my 'leg' hurts", when the pain is really in the thigh, may be similarly confusing.

2. Intensity

Any specific definition of pain should include the entire range of painful experience. That definition would have to encompass everything from the mild **intensity** of sensation of a papercut to the severe intensity of pain that could stop your breathing to make you pass out. If you have experienced a flu shot, childbirth, a migraine headache, a kidney stone or long-bone fracture, you can likely appreciate the differences in these painful experiences, although you may have difficulty putting it into words. Most physicians and medical professionals prefer that you rate your pain on a scale from 1-10, with "1" signifying mild or minimal pain and with "10" signifying the most severe pain.

Too often, patients with pain, rate their pain at a level of "10". Rating pain at this level is not usually helpful and may actually invalidate the level of your true pain. For example, "10" is the highest rating on this scale, and suggests that your pain is the highest that pain can be. If you however are able to be seen by a physician or nurse in a clinic setting, rather than being rushed to the hospital, then your provider may assume that the level you are giving is not credible. They may assume that you are magnifying your level of pain.

For that reason, it is best to define the intensity of your pain with deference to certain references that are relatable to all people. One of my patients, who had given a lot of thought to pain came up with this scale which I believe is comical, but very helpful:

She rates an "8" as the pain she would have if she was giving birth to a child without anesthesia. She rates a "9" as to what it would be like to be doused with gasoline then set on fire. She gives a "10" as what pain would be like if she was giving birth, while being set on fire, then having her eyebrows.

While obviously, this scale was created with a sense of humor, it is helpful in that it clearly references pain to situations that to most people are imaginable. Most pain that is evaluated in a non-emergent setting will be less that what women experience at the time of delivery. That being said, most pain that people are able to cope with prior to seeing a medical professional will be a "6" or "7" at most. People however feel that if they call their pain a level "2" or "3" that this may suggest that their pain is not significant or worthy of treatment. On the contrary, placing your pain level in the range of "2" to :5" suggests that your pain is not only real, but you have a realistic portrayal of your level. Where as the person who sits calmly in a doctors office, ambulates under their own power, and casually reads a magazine, is less credible when they state that their pain is a "10"

In addition, one of the ways health-care providers are able to assess how you are responding to treatment is by the changes in the level of intensity of your pain after treatment is instituted. For example, a person who is an '7" on his or her initial evaluation and then drops to a "4" is good evidence that their pain is responding to the medication or other treatment that has been started. Patients whose levels increase are ones for whom the instituted treatment has failed or ones who have experienced a change in the process leading to the pain. On the other hand, patients who present to the doctors initially with a "10", and report that their pain has worsened when they return on follow-up, it is harder to evaluate, since it is 'technically' impossible to have a pain worse than "10".

3. Acute vs Chronic Pain

The third way pain can be experienced, described or defined is through its relationship to time. Pain may be **acute**, which is usually defined by sudden onset but usually has a defined endpoint. The pain associated with a cut that heals in a 10 days or a sprain that heals in a few weeks is acute. **Chronic**

pain, on the other hand is pain that has been present for a period of time (usually 6 weeks or 6 months) and will likely persist for a long period of time, perhaps for more than 3 months to a lifetime. An example of chronic pain would be the pain of an ankle sprain or fracture that does not heal properly and leads to arthritis. Pain may also be defined as episodic, occurring over relative brief periods of time, like 'ice-pick' headaches

Sometimes, chronic pain begins with an acute pain episode. Back pain commonly begins this way, and when it fails to properly recover, turns into a chronic version that can be inconvenient or nearly completely disabling.

4. Quality of Pain

The third way to define your pain is by the quality of the pain you experience. Descriptors used to specify the quality of Pain include: dull, sharp, boring, burning, stabbing, pins & needle-like sensation, and tearing.

Phantom pain, the pain perceived in a limb or body part that has been amputated, is even harder to describe specifically.

5. Pain Progression

Lastly, pain may also be described in terms of its progression, whether it is worsening or improving with time. The importance of this being part of the definition helps to determine the natural history or course for the pain should it remain untreated and helps to guide the type of treatment itself.

Got it? With these descriptors you are armed and ready to define you pain specifically and you are now able to communicate to your health-care provider.

Chapter 3

How to Find a Doctor or other Health-care Provider to Treat your Pain

For example, what may seem to be an ankle-sprain injury following a twisting episode, may actually be a fracture that involves the ankle joint surface. Each can produce severe pain, lots of swelling and bruising, but a fracture involving the joint surface, if overlooked, may result in a chronic problem like arthritis. When arthritis affects the ankle joint, there may be significant pain with each step and every time you bear weight on that extremity. Once arthritis sets in following trauma, there are no easy treatment solutions. Injections may help, but they are most likely to provide temporary relief, and weaken the joint in other ways. In the long run, these injections may prove more harm than good. When the arthritis is severe, and the pain symptoms are unbearable, the only option may be an ankle fusion or an ankle joint replacement. Both surgical procedures are major. The ankle fusion will alter the way you walk, and inevitably lead to knee pain, back pain or both. Similarly, ankle joints may not last long, like artificial joint replacements of the hip and knee. The lack of longevity may beget other major surgery, which may be more difficult to perform than the original due to the loss of bone stock. Eventually, the only option that may remain is ankle fusion.

Odds are from the time your pain becomes chronic pain, you have a lot of time to think about it, to experience it, and to watch it effect its negative impact on the quality of your life. The relationships you have with people become impacted by your pain. During that time, you may question your own toughness and self-worth. You may beat yourself up. You may become depressed because you canny escape the pain you have. Other people in your life may sense your depressed mood, and may react in ways that only reinforce your sadness and hopelessness.

You can continue on the downward spiral of devastation, but before you reach the bottom, it makes sense to find a doctor/practitioner to treat your pain.

B. Finding the Right Doctor or Health-care Provider:

In the age of overwhelming expenses in medical care, the obtrusive interventions by insurance companies and managed-care plans, finding the doctor or health-care provider to evaluate and manage your pain may be bit confusing. Being a patient in a pain management clinic is not easy. There is a great demand for this type of care in the face of forces in every state to make it more difficult to have access to this care. The goal of this chapter is to help you find the right doctor and situation for you care, and to explain and demystify the process. Let me help you simplify the process.

1. **The Emergency Department (ED) or Emergency Room.**

The Emergency Department or Emergency Room is an important part of the health-care continuum. But they tend to be understaffed at times, high-stress environment, and surprisingly an environment that is not exactly kind to patients. It should be remembered that the ER is to be used for emergent and urgent medical situations and not as a substitute for a pain-management clinic.

People come to the ED for life and death situations, like heart attacks difficulty breathing, strokes, trauma. And the largest amount of resources will be relegated to helping patients with these situations. These people could die without the proper priority. If your pain level is the same as it was the previous week and month or year, it is not truly an emergency. And, the providers treating you in the emergency department will not treat your situation as an emergency. In fact, they may not treat you at all. More importantly, they may not treat your condition the way it needs to be treated.

In the ED, Patients typically report one of three types of reactions:

a. Under-treatment/Under-diagnosis. They are seen and cursorily evaluated. They get the feeling that are being treated as a "drug-seeker", or a person who is shopping around for medications who may not have a legitimate need for them, or their behavior is a part of larger problem of drug-addiction or drug-diversion. Drug diversion is the case where patients obtaining prescription medications that are typically controlled substances, and using the medication to sell or distribute in a criminal manner and for a recreational purpose. Because of the providers seeming ability to arrive at the wrong conclusion about your pain and your motivation for seeking care, they act defensively and offer little treatment while in the ED, and no treatment with pain medications upon your release, and recommending you follow up with your primary care practitioner. Patients with legitimate pain understandably feel insulted when they are treated in this manner. And Rightfully so. The doctor may secretly wish that you are sufficiently offended that you will never come back to that ED again.

b. Over-treatment/Under-diagnosis: They are seen and evaluated. But rather than a universal assessment of your pain, including its origins, there is a willingness by the doctor to prescribe medications for expediency. This may include a shot while you are in the ED or a prescription for medication, for the sole purpose of getting you out of the ED . This type of care is based on the principle when you are not in the ED, you are not their problem. For people with chronic pain, however, this is not a 'fix'. This is a 'band-aid' that only last until a few hours after the medication you were prescribed runs out.

c. Appropriate Treatment and Appropriate Diagnosis.   In this case, the patient presents to the ED with symptoms that the alert practitioner may recognize as an exacerbation of the usual level or baseline level of pain.   Following a careful examination, The physician then orders the appropriate diagnostic studies, which may include X-Rays, MRI and blood work to not only confirm diagnostic suspicions but to eliminate other diagnosis as causative for the presentation at the ED at the moment. For example, most people with 'bad backs' have 'bad backs', meaning chronically-strained muscles, degenerative disks or arthritis involving the joints of the back. Occasionally, the cause of the back pain or the change in the level of back pain may be not be as simple to explain. Especially, when that reason is something such as cancer which metastasizes or spreads to bones of the spine.   But if the physician never looks for this possibility, he or she will never find it. When they find it, it is too late. In the ED setting, with the demands of other patients with life-threatening conditions, the time it takes to do a careful work-up for back pain is not possible. But it it were, the goal after identifying the problem causing the pain is to set in motion a **treatment plan** to improve it. This could entail setting up follow-up care to manage the pain itself with a pain-management physician or with other providers including physical therapists, massage therapists, acupuncturists, and interventional physicians who can offer Epidural steroid injections, facet joint blocks and an evaluation by a surgeon if the problem is one which can be improved by surgery. Again, this level of care is beyond the scope of what can be provide through the ED.

In conclusion, if you must choose the Emergency Department, do so when it is clearly a matter of life or limb, and it is because a regular physician is not available to you. This will avoid what could be an unfruitful and unpleasant situation, that may not get you any closer to the treatment you need.

2. Your Family Doctor

a. What is a Family Doctor?

A family doctor is a doctor (MD or DO) who generally has specialized training in primary care or basic health-care, and the conditions that affect most people, children and adults. The term family doctor is based on the fact that can take care of each member of the family. Should your condition require more specialized care, they are able to contact and make referrals to other specialized physicians, such as internal medicine physicians (also known as *internists* who are specialists in systemic diseases like diabetes, high blood pressure problems, hospital-based medicine), orthopedic doctors (bone & Joint doctors), cardiologists (internal medicine sub-specialists who treat and diagnose heart conditions), general surgeons (abdominal surgeons), dermatologists (Skin doctors), rheumatologists (internists who sub-specialize in managing joint inflammation like that in Rheumatoid Arthritis, and Lupus), neurologists (managing strokes, brain and nerve disorders), oncologists (cancer treatment specialists) and other specialists and sub-specialists.

When speaking of "family doctor", occasionally other practitioners can and do perform similar duties. More and more, nurse practitioners (ARNP) are becoming a vital part of the health-care continuum. Like family doctors, they are well-suited to provide medical care and perform the functions of family medicine, independent of supervision by physicians. Nurse practitioners are registered nurses who have received additional training and certification in health-care, and have been a welcome solution to areas where the shortage of doctors cannot meet the demand of patients who need care. Other health-care providers include Physician Assistants, Nurses, Nursing Assistants, Medical Assistants but, in general, they require some degree of physician supervision. We use the term "Family doctor" in this handbook, although understanding that this role may be assumed by a Nurse practitioner, or another type of doctor with different specialized training who has agreed to serve the role of your primary care provider.

If you don't have a family doctor or primary care doctor, get one. It could be a matter of life and death, without you even knowing that it is. They may single-handedly save more lives or improve the outcomes than many other types of physicians. It is primarily through their annual examinations and evaluations of you that certain medical conditions may be found early. With early detection for many conditions, the outcomes are much more favorable. And in each age group, they can employ certain screening tests to check for the possibility of certain disease, like brain cancer and prostate conditions. Most other specialists are not equipped to have protocols in place for this type of screening. A doctor who has followed you for many years is more likely to be able to detect a change in you, even better than you may be able to. Also, having a family doctor is very help for the occasional health issues that occur sporadically that require treatment like colds, flu & rashes. Odds are that the treatment for non-emergent conditions and customer service you receive at your family physician are probably going to be superior to what you may received in an over-taxed emergency room.

b. The Ways to Find a Family Doctor

If you don't have a family doctor already:

1. Ask your friends,family and neighbors for their recommendations. This may be the best way to find a physician who can suit your needs.

2. If you have health insurance, call the customer service number and ask for the names of providers whose offices are close to you. Not all physicians accept all types of insurance, so it may be best to make sure that the physician is a provider under the insurance plan to make sure your visit will be

covered. Double-check with the physician's office you schedule the appointment to make sure he or she is a provider on that plan, or if not "In Network", your benefits will cover the visit.

3. Look in the Phone Book under Family Physician. Call a few of the offices, and explain your needs.

4. Call the nearest Chamber of Commerce. Although not all doctors will be listed here, you will be able to get some referrals for those that are close to you.

5. Google "Family Doctors"

6. Call your local Hospital. They will have a list of physicians who refer patients to this hospital or who treat and admit patients to this hospital.

7. Check the Newspaper for announcements of New Physicians to the area. Physicians who advertise in this manner are generally open to taking new patients.

8. Check with your **State Medical Association** or **State Medical Board** who maintain lists of active, licensed physicians in your area.

Just because you are able to find a family doctor doesn't guarantee that the doctor is accepting new patients. Established practices which desire to give quality care and good services may eventually become filled, so do not take it personally. If you find, the doctor's office cannot see you, then ask them if they have any recommendations for another physician who is accepting patients.

If you decide to use the internet for searches of your doctor, be careful. Some services like **HealthGrades**, **Yelp** or the **Better Business Bureau** are too often, simply billboards for disgruntled people to bash a doctor over reasons that are really not related to how good they are. For example, someone's dispute with a receptionist or staff member over a payment owed does not make any statement about the doctors ability to care for you. It is, however, a frequent motivation for that person to write a negative, scathing and unfair review for that doctor. Many of the reviews may not be true, or be ghostwritten by former employees, competitors, or other unqualified reviewers. Don't deny yourself a good doctor because of the "vandalism" you encounter on the internet that angry people resort to when they don't get their way.   You are smart. You can make the decision about the doctor you see when you meet him or her.

If you already have your family doctor, the process is so much easier. Your primary care doctor or family doctor is the place where your status of your health is known and where your medical history is warehoused. If your family doctor knows you well, then they may be both willing and qualified to treat your chronic pain.   In many ways, they will be more than qualified to treat you. They understand your allergies and sensitivities, and may have experience with other family members and may be able to make the correct recommendations for treating your pain, rather than starting from scratch, as you would do with a doctor who has never met you before. The disadvantage that some family doctors may have in treating your pain is that since pain is one of many conditions they treat, they may not be in the position to monitor you properly such that your treatment does not lead to unnecessary complications.   Primary care physicians may also not give the proper amount of respect to the differences in treating cute pain vs. chronic pain. Most health-care providers are capable of recognizing when they are not comfortable treating your pain. They may choose to monitor you for a period of time. If you fail to get better, or if they determine this is a problem that may be present for an extended period of time, then you will be better served by someone who specializes in managing pain.

In this case, they will refer you to a **pain-management specialist**, and will likely continue to care for your pain until you are able to be evaluated.

3. Finding a Pain-Management Specialist

Sometimes, even with a family doctor taking care of your basic health-care needs, you may still need to find a pain-management doctor on your own. In fact, more often you will need to do this that not. Your primary care doctor may not agree that you need one. Some doctors, believe it or not, don't 'believe in' pain management. They may not have personally experienced pain's debilitating effects on the body, psyche and soul. Don't feel bad about it if this is the reaction you encounter. Thank goodness, they have no idea what your pain is like!

Can you imagine how bad it would be if they had your level of pain?   You still have the right to get a second opinion, and to make the appointment yourself.

a. Here's how you find one:

1. Ask Your Friends or neighbors for their recommendations. Some of these people will have chronic pain, and may be able to make excellent recommendations, and may help you avoid pitfalls they may have encountered.

2. If you have health insurance, call the customer service number and ask for the names of providers whose offices are close to you. Again, not all physicians accept all types of insurance, so it may be best to make sure that the physician is a provider under the insurance plan to make sure your visit will be covered. Double check with the physician's office you schedule the appointment to make sure he or she is a provider on that plan

3. Look in the Phone Book under **Pain-management Physician**.   Or call your

local hospital for names and numbers. Call a few of the offices, and explain your needs.

4. Google "Pain Doctors" or "Pain-Management Doctors"

.

5.   Check with your State Medical Association or State Medical Board who maintain lists of active, licensed physicians in your area who practice pain management.

b. Other Things You Should Consider Once you find Your Pain-Management Doctor

Some of the considerations before you make your call is that the physician who you are trying to see may require a referral from another physician, ie your primary care provider, as a condition to see you as a patient. If your primary care doctor does not agree that you need to be seen by a pain doctor, then it may require that you "negotiate" with the primary care doctor's office, explaining that you would like to have a second opinion on your pain condition. If your primary care doctor still refuses, then you may have to find a new family doctor who may feel differently about your specific case or pain management, in general. This is like starting over, but it is probably for the best If you and the primary care physician you have chosen are not able to see eye-to-eye over something this basic, then it is worth a change.

There may also be some negotiation that is possible with the pain-management doctor you are trying to see. The doctor or staff member taking your call may be sympathetic to your plight, as they themselves understand that not all physicians have an appreciation for how important managing pain is for some patients. In this case, they may simply ask for your relative records and studies (like X-Rays, MRIs) that you may have had in the past, and have you come in.

With other pain-management practices, there may not be room for negotiation. A referral from another doctor may be an absolute requirement. Your insurance coverage may also mandate that you be referred in order for them to agree to cover it. You can verify which situation is applicable by calling customer relations for your insurance plan. The purpose of this rule may have in roots in the doctor trying to avoid seeing people who are truly drug-seeking and don't have a legitimate purpose in seeing the physician. To combat against the 'criminal' who uses the doctors visit, often paid for by their insurance policy, to obtain a prescription for narcotic medication, which in turn, may be diverted or sold to other people is clearly not a transaction that most physicians are willing to be part of. Moreover, a physician can pay dearly if he or she is found to not have safeguards in place, like referrals, to deter against this behavior. By mandating a referral from another doctor who has documented the presence of the pain, the pain doctor is making it harder for the system to be abused in this manner. Of course, this is not fool proof, by any means.

If there is no room for negotiation, simply call the next pain practice on your list. Eventually, you will be able to find a practice to accommodate you. I've personally encountered a number of hardworking, self-employed people in the construction business, who have pain from years of hard work, but due to expense, were not able to have regular follow-up with a family physician. Not addressing their worsening musculo-skeletal pain, however, threatens their ability to provide for themselves and their families. In these cases, they were able to find empathetic and welcoming providers to take care of them.   I feel you will be able to do the same.

4.   The Type of Pain-Management Doctor
There are more than one type of Pain Management doctors in terms of the services and expertise they can offer you . You will definitely need to make sure that you will be seeing the right type of pain-management doctor. The field of pain management is still quite young, unlike other many other medical specialties. Some doctors, **Medical Pain-Management Specialists**, focus on the management of pain primarily with conservative measures, including medications, joint injections, and trigger-point injections, but also employing a variety of other modalities like Physical Therapy, Massage Therapy, Water Therapy, and referrals to other practitioners, such as Chiropractors, Naturopathic Specialists, acupuncturists and other more-specialized pain doctors (see below).

A second type of pain-management specialists, **Interventional Pain-Management Specialists**, utilize interventional procedures to help improve pain. In general, these physicians may have specialty training in procedures that include Epidural Steroid Injections, Nerve blocks, Radio-frequency Nerve ablations, Pain Pump placement, Spinal Cord Stimulator implantation, Percutaneous disc procedures, Kyphoplasty or Vertebroplasty for Vertebral Compression Fractures due to Osteoporosis. Although their graduate medical training may include all of these procedures, they may opt to practice only selected procedures. Interventional Pain-management doctors generally receive referrals from primary care physicians and medical pain-management doctors. Patients do not generally refer themselves to this type of doctor, because an examination and evaluation of studies to identify the diagnosis needs to be made prior to going to the interventionalist.

A third type of pain-management physician is one who restricts his or her patients to a certain type of pain. For example in an oncology practice, there may be providers who treat pain in the context of cancer patients. Certain pain medicines are only FDA-approved for cancer patients. A provider of this type would allow the oncologist to treat the cancer itself, and permit the other provider to address the patients pain, which may be an important part of their quality of life. Other types of pain physicians restrict their practice to musculo-skeletal pain or orthopedic pain. Clearly, with the prevalence of back pain, a physician could spend all of the their time only treating this problem. Some physicians limit their practice to headaches. They are neurologists, typically. There are a number of pain centers in American where patients are referred exclusively for intractable headache pain and migraines.

5. Qualities that indicate a Good fit with your doctor:

Not all doctors are created equally. The one you find first, may not be the one who is best suited for you. Even if he or she is not perfect, the doctor still may provide you with acceptable and even exceptional care. A doctor may be friendly, but he or she is not your friend. He or she is the person you are hiring to take care of your pain in the safest way possible. Sometimes you may have a different view on things that are odds with what your doctor thinks. Remember, no matter how likable your doctor is, he is not a friend. His or her objective is to keep you comfortable, functional at the lowest level of medication possible to minimize the risk of toxicity to your organ systems, addiction, and the tolerance you body has to these medications.   To be effective, your provider must be an adequate listener, make you feel comfortable, provide a non-judgemental atmosphere, and provide clear and understandable plan for your treatment.

Let's review these qualities in depth:

i. Listening; Is the doctor a good listener. Listening to you is the key to communication. Communication is what allows the provider to detect whether or not there is a change or a new problem that may result in a change in your treatment. Not listening may cause the doctor to miss a critical clue that may cause you to suffer unnecessarily. If you think your doctor is not listening to you, then move on.

ii. Comfort : Do you feel comfortable with the provider. Do you feel un-rushed and un-hurried? Are you allowed to tell your story? Or, are you constantly being cut-off and redirected.   Some providers do have a habit of speaking fast and cutting the patients off mid-sentence, sometimes without even realizing it.   All it usually takes is a gentle request to permit you to finish your statements and to complete your thoughts , so that you can give the most accurate depiction of your pain. Most providers will graciously tone down their behavior, but do know, that they know what they are doing. They treat pain many times daily every day, and have an appreciation of almost every different scenario and variation of pain possible.   Cutting you off, although a little rude, is their way of trying to get to the diagnosis for you, and to come up with treatment pain to get you out of pain. In most cases, It will not take an hour to do this. Maybe a just a few minutes, a brief examination, and a review of your studies is all it will take.

iii. Trustworthiness: Do you feel like your provider is one that you can trust by their demeanor and the way they interact with you. If you don't feel that you can forge a bond of trust with your provider, you should find another. It may take a few or many interactions to develop the sense of trust. But if you never achieve the feeling of trust, you will blame yourself for not listening to your own instincts if down the line you realize that you should have never placed your trust in your provider.

iv.   Non-judgemental Atmosphere: Do you feel like you are being judged? Do you feel like you are being treated like "drug seeker" or drug addict.? Believe it or not, this would be unusual for a pain-management office. Everyone they see is expected to have a certain level of pain, unlike the population of patients seeing other type of physicians. Their awareness of people without a legitimate need for pain medications, who have only come in to abuse the medicines or divert them, is very high, although you may not recognize it. If you do feel like you are being judged in any way other that sympathy for the pain you are having, this may not be the right provider for you. Any other judgements of your motivation for seeking care for your pain does not provide a sound basis for a long-term relationship with your pain care provider.

v. A Clear and Understandable Treatment Plan: Does the treatment plan and diagnosis you are given by the provider make sense to you? Do you understand what your responsibilities as a patient are, specifically with regard to taking the medications, disposing of medications, reporting a reaction to the medication? Do you understand what is expected of you inf your pain becomes worse than what it has been while you are on the current treatment plan?   The answers to these questions should be clear in your mind at the conclusion of your first visit. If not, there could be bad problems down the line. Don't be afraid to ask questions. Don't hesitate to call the doctors office to ask questions if they arise.

Chapter 4

Understanding Your Evaluation and Treatment Plan

Once you find a doctor that you believe can help you and one that you are comfortable with, the doctor will formulate a treatment plan for your pain, after the your evaluation. Your evaluation will consist of your "history" and performance of a physical exam. If you had have previous studies, the doctor will likely want to review them or know their results. Then, there may be studies that the doctor orders which may better help define your pain and its potential for successful treatment.

A. What is an History?

The History is the part of your visit where the physician identifies your problem, or what is bothering you or the reason for your visit in a general manner.

1. Chief Complaint

The history begins with your **"Chief Complaint"**. It does not mean you are a 'Complainer'. It is just what the portion of this evaluation is called. Examples of common Chief Complaints that are encountered in the pain-management clinic include:

"My Back Hurts"

"I have pain traveling down the back of my leg"

"I have frequent headaches"

"My Knee is painful and swells"

2.   History of Present Illness (HPI)

Once Identified, the doctor will elicit the 'story' behind your chief complaint, called the **"History of Present Illness" (or HPI)**. He or she may begin getting this story by asking you questions like

How long has it bothered you or "When did this problem start?". For some people, Communicating the story behind a medical problem is not easy. The doctor is trained for this possibility and will piece together the story with you by asking more questions. Some patients are very good 'historians', who in telling their 'story' can recall the exact moment their pain started and the progression of the pain over time leading to the visit. It is also okay if you don't know when things began, as sometimes pain comes on insidiously.

The doctor's HPI that is constructed from your visit will contain some, if not all, of the following answers to these questions:

When did the pain begin?

How do you rate the severity of your pain on a pain scale?

Was the pain onset related to trauma or an accident?

Has your pain changed over time?

What makes it better and What makes it worse?

Does it travel?

Do you have family members with similar pain?

If you have seen other doctors, what was the diagnosis you were given?

Have you had any X-rays or other studies done? What were the results?

What kind of treatment have you had for this pain? Did it help?

3.   Past Medical History

The doctor will then explore your **Past Medical History**. Some of this may have already been provide to him through your initial paperwork you filled out or from questions that the doctors assistant or nurse has asked you. The PMH is basically a list of your past and present medical conditions that you have including Hypertension (High Blood Pressure), Diabetes, Heart problems, Asthma, Breathing or Lung Problems, Cancer you have or have had, Hepatitis, HIV, and genetic conditions you were born with.   The importance of the doctor knowing about your conditions and documenting them is because his or her decisions about your treatment, what studies are appropriate and what medications are appropriate may depend on this information.

4. Past Surgical History

The doctor will then ask you about your previous surgeries, or **Past Surgical History**, as it may also guide treatment decisions and decisions about diagnostic studies you can have. For example, some aneurysm surgeries, abdominal surgeries and back surgeries which involve the use of certain metals, clips or stimulators implanted deeply in the body are not suitable, and could be frankly dangerous for MRI procedures. The magnetic force of the MRI would cause severe heating and movement of the metal that could be catastrophic. Other surgical procedures, like back fusion surgery may give insight into and have implications for the pain you have now.

5. Allergies

The doctor will need to know your **Allergies**. She will review what medications, foods and substances you may have sensitivities to or allergic reactions to. This information is obviously important to make sure to avoid the use of medications that may trigger a reaction that may be life-threatening.

6. Review of Systems

The next area that the doctor will explore is the **Review of Systems**, a checklist of symptoms or signs of system function or dysfunction that may expand or minimize diagnostic possibilities. You may have filled out a checklist previous to seeing the provider that asked if you had any double-vision, eye redness, coughing, shortness-of-breath, difficulty swallowing, joint swelling, numbness, difficulty urination, skin irritation or rash, diarrhea, constipation, painful urination, bloody urine, frequent urination, etc.

7. Use of Substances

Usually following this time, the provider will ask you about your consumption of substances. Specifically tobacco products, alcohol products, and illicit substances. This information is not (or really should not) be used to judge your behavior, but rather to give diagnostic clues about your pain problem, and to determine your relative risk of addiction or abuse of substances. It is important to answer these questions accurately and truthfully. Lying or misleading your doctor will injure the doctor-patient relationship, perhaps irreparably.

a. Tobacco Products. The risk of lung cancer and oral cancer with tobacco products has been well-established. He effect of smoking on back pain is also well-known. Smoking impairs the small-vessel circulation in the body.   The disks in the spine are particularly vulnerable to this impairment, and if disks become injured, the lack of sufficient blood supply from the small vessels of the neighboring bone surfaces will result in a predictable, irreversible degeneration of the disks over time. Alcohol can be important particularly for its effect on the metabolism, of drugs by the liver, the health of the liver, and the risk of harm that may occur when pain medications are taken concurrently with the alcohol. If alcohol abuse is suspected by the physician, this will definitely have implications on the type of treatment that would be recommended.

b. Illicit Substances

Illicit substances are also noted by the physician. Again, it is important to be accurate and honest about your consumption. Many people feel the need to conceal their use of these substances out of fear that they may be judged as a "bad" person or they will be turned in to law enforcement if the y admit their use.   To the contrary, the physician's primary role is not to "turn you over to law enforcement", rather it is to determine whether or not your use of this substance represents a threat to your health and safety. All clinics and providers will approach the problem of illicit use differently. There will also be variations by State and regions of the country. There may be different policies based on different substances, particularly **marijuana.**

c. Marijuana

In some states, Marijuana is legal for medical purposes only, including some painful conditions. There are also clinical studies validating the benefit of Marijuana in the treatment of pain. In other states, marijuana is legal for medical use and recreational use. This means for the pain patient who consumes marijuana 'legally', your provider will be able to make recommendations about pain medicine with deference to your marijuana use, so that it will be safe for you.

In states like my own, Marijuana is not classified as a legal substance for recreational purposes or for medical use. For pain management in States like this one, it is advisable to quit smoking marijuana as a condition of treatment, as the physician cannot defend or condone the use of a medicine that illegal by the state granting him or her the license to practice. If a patient is harmed, and the physician knowing neglects the use of marijuana, the physician may be liable for the patients harm in a court-of-law. In my experience, most patients, actually almost all, who consume marijuana on a recreational basis, would give it up to have the chance to have adequate pain control. Those who have consumed it for a period of 20-years or more on a daily basis may have difficulty quitting . Patients in this category may require a weaning process. Even still, the levels of marijuana as indicated by urine testing will persist for several weeks after they have quit. Some patients, no matter the level of pain they have, will never give up using this substances. Some clinics may elect to ignore this by not testing for its presence in urine samples . Others may decide that the patient is not a suitable candidate for pain management, solely because it is an illicit substance. Hopefully, the change in attitudes, social morays, and legislation will result in a unification in policy that will permit consistency in the treatment of patients who need this substance or just simply enjoy using this substance.

As a matter of truth and science, Marijuana has been shown to positively improve pain control in patients, and has not been shown to be as dangerous in terms of death and injury as alcohol, which is a legal substances. It may also be safer than most prescription drugs.

d. Other Illicit Substances

With other substances, like Methamphetamine, Heroin, Cocaine, Methadone (when not prescribed by a physician), Ecstasy, PCP, etc, the same assumptions that we make for Marijuana do not apply. In general, these substances cause a greater degree of mental impairment and compromise, and have a higher potential for abuse and addiction than Marijuana does. So, patients who acknowledge use of these substances need to be screened carefully, as prescribing them pain medicines may not be justifiable, even though they may have pain. Many physicians will outright refuse to prescribe narcotic medications or controlled substances to any patient with a recent history of use of these illicit medications. Certainly, if you deceive the physician about your use, and the substances then appear in your urine test, then the relationship between you and the doctor is nullified and, for your safety and best interests, no narcotic medication will be prescribed. The condition upon which these medications are prescribed to you is "Trust". You can never violate this condition with these medications. Ever.

A patient who acknowledges challenges with these illicit substances is best referred back to their referring physician for further guidance and help with substance abuse. If this is not possible, the pain-management physician usually has a list of other physicians who specialize in addiction and abuse who can help the patient overcome this challenge.

Having a past history of substance abuse, does not necessarily preclude treatment for pain management. The practice of medicine is based on being "humane". Clearly people who have had a history of substance of abuse can also have pain that requires treatment. Substance abuse does not nullify that history. The physician may agree to treat you but want to monitor you more carefully to make sure there are no relapses. If you have this problem, doing this is not punishment. It is for your safety and protection.

B. Radiographic Studies

1. Xrays:

Common studies that may be considered are X-rays, an imaging technique or radiographic study with which you are probably familiar. In some cases. this can be done as a part of your visits in the doctors office. They may reveal important things about your bones, joints and how they relate to each other. Some inferences may be made about the soft tissues (non-bone structures) based on the faint shadows they may produce. Arthritis, for example, the degenerative (or 'wear-or-tear) form or the inflammatory kind (e.g. Rheumatoid Arthritis) have suggestive patterns that can be recognized on X-Ray fairly easily. Spine X-rays can also reveal degenerative patterns which may be helpful in treatment and may also reveal information about the condition of the disks, the shock-absorbing cushions between the vertebral levels, to determine their state. Sometimes, rare causes of pain, possibly warranting special treatment, can be identified by X-rays. For example, evidence of a genetic condition known as *Ankylosing Spondylitis* (AS), a rare form of back pain and joint pain, may be identified by X-rays. *Spondylolysis*, a condition characterized by a defect in the posterior part of spin bones can also be identified with special views on X-rays. Identifying the condition correctly will result in more rapid, efficient and effective treatment of these conditions with the help of the Rheumatologist, (for AS), and the Spine Surgeon (for Spondylolysis).

There are many other reasons that X-rays can not only be helpful, but crucial. An even more rare finding on X-rays is the finding of tumors in bones or evidence of cancer that is spreading or metastatic, that can lead to the proper treatment course. Sometimes, pain that is experienced in the back is actually due to an aneurysm in the abdominal level of the Aorta. Evidence of enlargement and calcification of this vessel that is visible on an X-ray may be the first indication that this condition needs to be addressed. Back pain occurring because of kidney stones is sometimes discovered on X-rays serendipitously. You would be amazed at the number of times 'simple back pain' is treated without radiographic studies for months, and the cause turns out to be something potentially deadly, like cancer or an Abdominal Aortic Aneurysm on the verge of rupture.

X-rays may not be sufficient to delineate the problem completely from the diagnostic and management perspective. For example for abdominal pain patients, X-rays may provide little benefit in a diagnostic sense, unless the pain is acute. Acute pain in the abdomen is sometimes associated with abnormal gas patterns which may signify the need for surgery. For chronic abdominal pain , this is probably not as helpful outside of calcification of the gallbladder. Similarly, X-rays of the head probably will not reveal a lot substantively helpful information about headaches and migraine pain.

2. MRI, CT Scan and Ultrasounds:

MRIs, CT scans, and Ultrasounds are the second line studies beyond x-rays that your doctor may order to investigate possibilities of diagnoses that underlying your pain.

a. MRI

MRI is Magnetic Resonance Imaging. It is a very useful technology that allows reconstruction of areas of the body without invasiveness. The Radiologist is able to examine the films which consist of multiple images arranged as sequential 2-dimensional slices, representing sections of an area of a body a few millimeters apart. The radiologist will interpret these images, knowing what is 'normal' and what is 'not normal', so that your primary doctor or pain-management specialist can correlate the findings and develop ideas regarding your true diagnosis. If you looked at these images, and you could stack each individual image slice on each other, you could be able to visualize the body area as if you could see through the body in 3 dimensions. The ability of a structure in the body to produce a signal on MRI is determined by its water content. The images are not in color, but they are presented on a grey scale. Contrast, provided through a vein or orally, will allow illumination of certain structures in better detail. For example, the vessels and organs which contain a high density of vessels or vasculature (like the liver and bone marrow) show up brightly with IV contrast. The use of contrast may be the only way to identify certain disorders or pathology. To image the stomach and intestines, contrast provided by mouth ahead of time makes it possible to identify abnormalities that may be leading to pain or illness.

The MRI study is usually done at an outside facility or hospital radiology department. The radiation the magnet emits is not harmful, like the radiation of X-rays has the potential to be. If you are pregnant or have certain types of surgically-implanted hardware, wound staples or retained metal from a gunshot or penetrating injury, you may be excluded from having this study done due to safety concerns. The machines are usually too expensive to be part of a single doctor's office. The procedures have a schedule they follow, so it is important when you are scheduled to be there ahead of time to fill out paperwork and to provide any insurance information, if that has not already been done prior to your arrival. It may be appropriate for you to avoid eating or drinking for a period of time before the study, but don't expect this to be the case, unless you were told otherwise. The procedure will take anywhere from 20 minutes to hours, depending on the area or areas to be studied. You will be placed on a platform that inches its way into a tunnel the magnet area of the machine. It will be noisy and sometimes headphones playing music will be provided to you. It is important to remain completely still and breathe as directed by the radiology assistant, so that the clearest, most crisp images will be possible. If you discover that you are claustrophobic or having a fear of tight spaces that cannot be overcome, other arrangements, like providing you with sedation, or rescheduling your study for an open-MRI, which provides less of a constricting environment may be done.

In general, the results of the MRI will be read within 24-48 hours and the written report will be faxed or mailed to your doctors office prior to your next visit. In situations where a cancer, unstable fracture, infection or other serious unforeseen diagnosis is encountered, it is common practice for the radiologist to contact the primary doctor ordering the study immediately to report this results, so that an intervention may be made. Many of the radiology technicians are well-trained in which circumstances to call the radiologist to view an abnormal finding that warrants immediate attention. So, if you have just had a study, and you receive a call from your doctors office shortly thereafter, then you know that you should respond urgently. If you do not get a call, in most cases, it is safe to assume that your diagnosis does not involve a life-or-death type of emergency.

b. CT Scans

A CT scan is also called computerized tomography. The images developed from this study are displayed in a manner similar to MRI scan films. The radiation used to compute and reconstruct the images in CT scanning are X-rays, so pregnancy is usually a contraindication for having this study done out of concern for the fetus. The set-up for A CT scan is similar, but the tunnel is much wider, but no-so-much so that claustrophobic patients will be comfortable. Some problems leading to pain may be better suited for analysis by CT scan, rather than MRI scan. Certain body structures, like bones, are easy to analyze by CT scans, because the technology is based on x-rays. Conversely, the organs and soft-tissues are hard to image by CT, unless they are calcified. Special contrast dye can be used orally or intravenously to assist in enhancing the imaging by CT so that other structures can be more easily identified. For some back problems, specifically ones that occur following surgical treatment, Imaging is best done using dye that injected directly into the spinal fluid. This study is called a CT-Myelogram. For other patients with previous back surgery, who, because of implants that are susceptible to magnetization, may not be candidates for an MRI, but can be candidates for CT scanning or CT-myelography.

As with MRI studies, emergent results will be reported to your physician immediately.

c. Ultrasounds and other studies.

Occasionally , Ultrasounds may be used to assess an area. This is common for blood clots in the leg leading to swelling and pain, for which a specific Ultrasound technique can readily identify. Ultrasounds are also useful in evaluating pain that originates in organs, like testicular pain & gall bladder pain. EMG (electro-myography) and Nerve conduction studies can help identify conditions involving nerves as in nerve damage (neuropathy) and may be able to pin pint where the nerve issue is located in the spine (radiculopathy) or there is entrapment somewhere along the arm, wrist (carpal tunnel) or leg. Many other special or 'non-routine' studies may be considered in the course of diagnostic evaluation that are ordered on the basis of the specific symptoms and signs that the patient shows.

C. Blood work

Blood testing may or may not be routine for an initial evaluation by your pain-management doctor. But there are clearly circumstances which may warrant basic testing. If there is any concern of your general health status, basic chemistries (Sodium, potassium, bicarbonate, chloride, glucose, Blood Urea Nitrogen (BUN) and Creatinine) and blood counts (hemoglobin, hematocrit, platelets and white blood cell count with differential) should be done. Abnormalities in these values may require a more stringent medical evaluation by a primary care physician or internist, to avoid health consequences and to treat diagnoses that are unrelated to the pain. They may also correct abnormalities that could impact or amplify pain. An expanded chemistry panel may be done to assess liver baseline values, which may change in an unwanted and unexpected direction after commencement of treatment with certain medications. Elevation in liver enzymes, known as AST and ALT, may demand additional testing to determine the presence of hepatitis, which may foster the opportunity for treatment of this condition. Further, it will allow the least harmful medication for pain to chosen so as not to aggravate the vulnerable organ system. Also, the baseline values may be helpful in the initial institution of therapies when the impairment of the liver or kidney is already known.

Other blood tests, like the may indicate the status of other organs. Elevated amylase enzymes may be consistent with pancreatitis, which can be a source of apparent back pain or abdominal pain. Calcium levels may help assess whether there are problems with Calcium metabolism affecting the skeletal system, which may be altered in women after menopause who are at risk for osteoporosis. Elevated Muscle enzymes, creatine kinase, or muscle breakdown products like Myoglobin, in the blood or urine may signify a inflammatory condition that is destroying the muscle, as is common with forms of myositis.

Blood work may also be obtained when **rheumatological (or inflammatory) conditions** are suspected. The ESR (erythrocyte sedimentation rate or "Sed rate"), along Test for Rheumatoid Factor, C-reactive protein, ANA (anti-nuclear antibody), anti-phospholipid antibody, anti-doublestrand DNA antibodies, HLA-B27, HLA-DR4, uric acid and others. These tests may aid in the diagnosis of any of a multitude of rheumatologic or autoimmune-related conditions including Rheumatoid Arthritis, Systemic Lupus Erythematosus, Ankylosing Spondylitis, Reiter's Syndrome, Sjogrens Syndrome, Psoriatic Arthritis, Behcet's Disease. Elevations in uric acid, hyperuricemia, are consistent with Gout and will assist in controlling the symptoms of gout, including "gouty arthritis". Positive values in your blood work do not necessarily 'confirm' a diagnosis. But in a good percentage of cases, they help establish the correct diagnosis. Confirmation of positive values along with signs consistent with a rheumatological condition warrant an evaluation by a **Rheumatologist**. The treatments they can offer are highly-specialized and are not available through other physicians in some cases. The treatment they prescribe as in the case of Rheumatoid Arthritis may modify the disease's aggressiveness so that the risk of joint deformities can be minimized for some patients. The waiting time to see a rheumatologist can be long, as they are few in number, and patients tend to be with these doctors for a lifetime. Your pain-management doctor is usually happy to treat your pain symptoms until you are able to see the rheumatologist.

Outside of the initial testing, your pain-management doctor may order blood work to be done at 4- to 6-month intervals, to make sure your liver and kidney function are stable with your prescribed treatment.

D. Formulation of Your Treatment Plan

Based on your evaluation and your studies your doctor will develop an Impression of your Diagnosis or the diagnostic possibilities and will formulate a treatment plan. Because you are unique, your treatment plan will be customized. Certain parts of the plan, however, may be predictable.

1. Observation

On the basis of your evaluation, the doctor may decide to 'observe' you for a period of time to get a better feel of what your pain is like, how frequently it occurs. It is very likely that since you are referred to the pain specialist, other providers have already done this. This step may not be needed. Other pain-specialist do this routinely.

2. Conservative Treatment

There are several conservative strategies that can be employed in the treatment of pain.

a. Physical Therapy:

Physical Therapy, consisting of strengthening and stretching of muscles under the supervision of a trained therapist, is a well-established way of treating painful conditions. They can also provide a rehabilitation and conditioning program for parts of the body which facilitate a return to normal activity and function. There are also "modalities" that physical therapist can apply like Ultrasound therapy, Electrical Stimulation (TENS unit, Interferential Devices) and Heat and Cold therapy that may also be helpful in reducing pain. Typically, patients see the therapist 2- 3 times-a-week for up to 6 weeks, although the schedule may vary. With the approval of your referring doctor, the schedule may continue so long as a benefit is appreciated and progress is being made. A home program may also be prescribed upon completion of the physical therapy so that your progress will continue.

The initial visit with the therapist will also involve an evaluation and assessment, so that the best approach to treating your condition can be chosen. Some patients clearly benefit from these treatments. Some do not. Some peoples pain actually worsen as a result of Physical Therapy. Under this circumstance, it should be discontinued.

b.   Massage Therapy

On occasion, massage therapy may be recommended. The precise mechanism by which therapeutic massage improves pain is not clear. However, many patients find comfort and relief from this type of treatment, which is the reason it is commonly utilized.   There are many massage techniques that may be employed. Some find Deep Tissue Massage, Trigger Point Pressure/Acupressure, and Rolfing (soft-tissue manipulation) good ways to get relief of tight, spasm-ridden, painful areas. Others may prefer the more gentle massage techniques like Swedish for relief of pain and relaxation.   In a general sense, Massage is believed to stimulate circulation in the muscles and tissues, and to facilitate lymphatic circulation and drainage, which helps eliminate toxins in the body which may aggravate pain.

Massage does not help everyone. Massage is not always affordable for everyone. There is no specific schedule guidelines that are written in stone, but many massage therapists will recommend weekly massages until the pain is better controlled. More frequently than this, particularly with the more intensive types of massage, may cause damage to muscles and soft-tissues.

c.   Chiropractic Manipulation

On occasion, chiropractic treatment involving manipulation for pain relief may be suggested. Some allopathic (MD)and osteopathic (DO) physicians believe in the value of manipulation for the improvement of certain conditions that involve pain and they may suggest or refer patients for this type of treatment. The number of patients who swear by the chiropractic physician is a testimony to the belief that this care is helpful. Other physicians may believe otherwise. The choice to have treatment by your chiropractor can be yours alone. If you are undergoing manipulations but not experiencing the improvement you expect, you may also choose to discontinue that treatment and avoid unnecessary expense. Some people also worry that chiropractic manipulation can be harmful somehow or that manipulation of the spine can result in paralysis. As one or more chiropractors have noted, more people are paralyzed by surgery of the spine than by chiropractic manipulation.

d. Water Therapy

Water therapy or hydrotherapy is a form of physical therapy that takes advantage of the many properties of water, such as its temperature and ability to facilitate buoyancy. Patients can use to water, in a pool for example, to perform exercises that may not be as safe outside of water due to falling. Water aerobic classes are a great example of the utility of hydrotherapy in building strength, facilitating mobility and stamina. It is a great way to rehabilitate and condition the body in a controlled fashion. Also, the presence of water surrounding the body, facilitates blood vessel smooth-muscle relaxation or contraction (vasodilation and vasoconstriction) depending on the temperature. Water in a whirlpool or jacuzzi environment can also provide relaxation and stimulate circulation in the muscles and tissues in a manner analogous to massage therapy.

e. Acupuncture

Acupuncture is a treatment that originated in ancient China, which involves the placement of fine needles through the skin at specific points (meridians, acupuncture points) to achieve pain reduction. Acupuncture is also used to treat other conditions that do not necessarily involve pain. The needles may be be placed alone or they may be connected to a device which produces an electrical stimulation.   Clinical analysis of this treatment has not demonstrated a significant benefit in the treatment of pain in the short-term or long-term, but there are many patients who swear by it. In most case the needle sticks are virtually painless, and the risks of adverse events are small.   Rarely, people may develop complications like skin infections, and even more rarely, pneumothorax (collapsed lung). All acupuncturist should use single-use needles to avoid the transmission of infection. This is something you should ask about before you consent to treatment.

f. Hypnosis

Many people consider hypnosis in the theatrical forms that you've heard of where audience members are selected, placed under a 'hypnotic spell' with a pendulum, and end up quacking like a duck. In reality, hypnosis, a technique that involves producing a deep state of relaxation through which suggestion can be made to the conscious and subconscious to modify behaviors or modify the level of pain is a credible way to improve pain. There are studies, albeit involving small numbers of patients and without controls, that have suggested that hypnosis can be useful in moderating pain levels. It is also clear that not every patient will be susceptible to 'hypnotic' suggestion. Additionally, the sessions can also be expensive.

g. Cognitive Behavioral Therapy

In its simplest definition, Cognitive behavioral therapy is an approach which modifies the impact the mind and behaviors have on pain. It utilizes techniques which help break the pattern of unhelpful thoughts, responses to stressors, and other behaviors which have influence the level or occurrence of pain.

3. Medical Management of Pain

On the basis of your level of pain and its impairment of your function and reduction of your quality of life, the doctor will likely recommend or prescribe medication for you pain. Many providers who treat pain, will use The **World Health Organization (WHO)** recommendations as a guide to treatment. The WHO 'Pain Ladder' provides a 3-step approach to the treatment of pain. The classes of pain they use are **mild, mild-to-moderate** and **moderate-to-severe**. If a patient is not responding sufficiently in one treatment class, then they are moved in a higher step on the treatment. Obviously, treatment must be individualized and customized, because in the difference that exist among people with pain.

In general,

Mild pain

can be treated with over-the-counter medications like acetaminophen (Tylenol) or Ibuprofen.

Mild-to-Moderate pain

Can be treated with Acetaminophen with or without Tramadol (Ultram)

Can also be treated with An opioid medication in combination with Acetaminophen, like Norco, Vicodin, or Percocet.

Moderate-to-Severe pain

Primarily with Opiates, Opioids, and their short-acting versions, Long-acting versions or combinations.

a. Over-The-Counter Pain Relievers

There are a variety of medications that can be taken over-the-counter, or purchased from your pharmacy or pharmacy-section of your grocery/department store without needing a prescription.

Aspirin (Bayer, St. Joseph)

Acetaminophen (Tylenol)

Arthritis Strength Tylenol (Time-released Acetaminophen)

Ibuprofen (Advil, Motrin)

Naproxen (Aleve)

Acetaminophen and Aspirin (Excedrin, Vanquish)

Acetaminophen and Diphenhydramine (Percogesic, Tylenol PM)

Aspirin and Caffeine (BC Powder)

Acetaminophen, Aspirin and Caffeine (Goody's Powder)

Many if not all of these medications are probably well-known to you and your family members. You are probably aware of how effective these medications are or have been on the pain you experience. You may not be aware of the mechanisms as to how they control pain. You may not also be aware of the risks that you take when you use these medications. "Over-the-counter" does not mean always safe or without risk. We will discuss these medication types.

Aspirin is a fever-reducing medication and an anti-inflammatory medication. The effect of anti-inflammatory agents on pain is to reduce the inflammatory (swelling, redness and heat) components that lead to pain or that worsen a painful incident. Certain nerves that conduct pain stimuli can also be regulated by a type of biologically-active chemical class or hormones called prostaglandins. The inhibition of the synthesis of specific prostaglandins can effect how a nerve transmits a pain signal, as certain nerve cells contain receptors on their surface which are capable of binding the hormone, and producing a specific response in these nerve cells. So in some cases, blocking the inflammation response by the medication can lessen the amount of pain you have. Aspirin may also have side-effects that are not tolerable or are dangerous. Aspirin impairs the ability of platelets in the blood to aggregate properly, which may lead to prolonged bleeding. Aspirin also interferes with the stomach linings ability to protect itself against acid erosion, causing stomach irritation (gastritis) and stomach ulcers. The ulcers combined with the deficient blood clotting capacity can mean large volumes of blood are lost through the gastrointestinal tract, which is responsible for many deaths and hospitalizations each year.

Ibuprofen is also an anti-inflammatory medication. Along with the over-the-counter medication **Aleve**

(and many other Prescriptive-medications), Ibuprofen is classified more specifically as a **non-steroidal anti-inflammatory drug (NSAID)**. The distinction between NSAIDs and the subclass of steroids which block inflammation, like prednisone, hydrocortisone and solumedrol, is that these medicine must be used sparingly, otherwise they begin to have unintended effects on other systems like bone mineralization, skin integrity, joint integrity, and the immune system integrity. The NSAIDs have structural similarity with aspirin, and similar mechanism of actions in their ability to reduce inflammation and pain, and similar side-effects and risks. In general, they are distinguished from each other in the doses needed to achieve the therapeutic effect, duration that it lasts in the body, the potency they may have and the degree of side-effects they cause.

Caffeine, the component used in some preparations, is a central nervous system stimulant, may assist pain-relief through increasing the absorption rate of the pain medicine, and by influencing the tone (constriction/dilation of the blood vessels) through its action as a hormone. This is why caffeine is a frequent formulation of headache medication preparations.

Diphenhydramine, also known as **Benadryl**, is a member of the class of drugs known as 'anti-histamines', which are used in the treatment of allergies. It has a side-effect of causing sedation and relaxation, which may improve pain by providing an escape that only relaxation and sleep can provide. There is also evidence that the histamine can modulate the pain response, independent of its ability to make you rest.

b. Prescription Medications

There are a variety of medication for 'mid-to-moderate' and 'moderate-to-severe' pain that your physician may prescribe for you. Most are based on the structure of morphine, which is an opiate, a chemical substance that is found in nature produced from extracts from the Opium Poppy plant. The family of naturally-occurring opiates and medications that are their chemically-Synthesized derivatives and analogues are called Opioids.

Not all opioid medications are natural substances, however. Not all opioid medications are legal substances. Both Codeine and Heroin, for example, are both derivatives of Morphine, but only Codeine is legal when it is prescribed by a doctor. Heroin is not legal or illicit.

Whereas it is beyond the scope of this book to provide the decision-making basis for using certain medications, and not others, we will present a list of commonly prescribed opioid medications. Factors related to the level of your pain, your medication allergies and sensitivities, and your liver/kidney function are part of the decision-making process. Other factors that will be considered are, the other medications you take that may interfere with potential medication that are chosen, your experience with previous pain medications, your tolerance to certain medications, any prior history of substance abuse or potential. It is also likely the providers comfort level with certain medications, and your ability to understand the instructions with medications will all be factors in that choice of medication will also be given consideration. Once the choice is made, the dose you are prescribed and the number that you are prescribed for a particular time-interval will be determined. Any questions as to why certain medications are prescribed for you should be addressed with your provider.

In a very general manner the medications listed become more powerful as you descend this list.

List

i. Oral Medications

Codeine

Codeine with Acetaminophen (Tylenol #3, Tylenol #4)

Dihydrocodeine with Acetaminophen and Caffeine (Trezix)

Hydrocodone

Hydrocodone, Extended release (Zohydro ER)

Hydrocodone with Acetaminophen (Norco, Vicodin, Lortab, Lorcet)

Hydrocodone with Ibuprofen (Vicoprofen, Reprexain)

Oxycodone (Roxicodone)

Oxycodone with Aspirin (Percodan)

Oxycodone with Acetaminophen (Percocet, Endocet, Tylox, Xodol)

Oxycodone, Extended Release (Oxycontin)

Oxycodone with Acetaminophen, Extended Release (Xartemis)

Meperidine (Demerol, Meperitab)

Morphine

Morphine, Extended Release (MSContin, Avinza Kadian)

Morphine with Naltrexone (Embeda)

Hydromorphone (Dilaudid)

Oxymorphone (Opana)

Oxymorphone, Extended Release (Opana ER)

Tapentadol (Nucynta)

ii. Transdermal Medications (Patches) for Extended Pain Control.

Fentanyl (Duragesic)

Buprenorphine (Butrans)

iii.   Nasal Spray

Butorphanol (Stadol) primarily for headache pain.

iv.   Other Pain Medications

Certain medications, namely **Subutex, Suboxone** and **Methadone** are used in pain management, they are usually not first-line choices for medications. They are also used, and mainly used, in the treatment of addiction to heroin and oxycodone, which is completely different than pain management.

vi.   Non Pain Medications used in pain management

There are a variety of medications which help in the management of pain which are not themselves pain medicines

Muscle Relaxers

Cyclobenzaprine (**Flexeril**), Tizanidine (**Zanaflex**), Metaxalone (**Skelaxin**), Orphenadrine (**Norflex**), Methocarbamol (**Robaxin**), Baclofen,

Chlorzoxazone(**Parafon Forte**), Diazepam (**Valium**) and Carisoprodol (**Soma**)

The muscle relaxers all work in different ways, and do not represent a single structural or biochemical class of medications. Care must be taken when prescribing Valium, a member of the benzodiazepine family. If a patient has been on this medicine at high-doses for prolonged period of time, detoxification in a hospital setting may be required if it is discontinued. Soma must also be prescribed and taken with care. One of its breakdown productions in the body can be toxic over time and is a well-known tranquilizer, that can increase sedation when no additional sedation is desired or desirable.

Nerve Medication:

Gabapentin (**neurontin**) and pregabalin (**Lyrica**) medications which can be used when there is associated nerve pain or such nerve symptoms as numbness, tingling and burning. There are also other medications which may have dual roles as anti-depressants and in controlling peripheral nerve pain like amitryptiline (**Elavil**) and duloxetine (**Cymbalta**) that can be prescribed.

Sleep Medication:

A subset of patients with pain will experience insomnia or difficulty sleeping,. This may be a temporary problem or one that is long-term. It may occur because there is pain. It may occur independent of the pain or may have pre-dated the chronic pain problem, but interferes with the ability to control pain. And, in some cases, the pain may be a result of the pain medicines themselves. Sleep studies and **Oximetry testing**, which checks the oxygen level s in your blood during sleep, are tests that your provider may order to help guide the treatment of the insomnia.

Thankfully, over-the-counter medications like Benadryl and herbal supplements Melatonin, Valerian, and L-Tryptophan are able to help a large number of people. Occasionally, medications like Zolpidem (**Ambien**) or Eszoplicone (**Lunesta**), may be used. Anti-depressants such as Cymbalta and Lyrica, can be used as well to facilitate sleep, and very importantly for patients who also have peripheral nerve pain and/or depression. Members of the benzodiazepine class like Valium, Xanax (alprazolam), Klonopin (clonazepam) can also be used, but only with caution, particularly since other medications that may be used may also cause sedation and depress respiration (the ability to breathe).

Chapter 5

Your Responsibilities

Pain management is more of a privilege these days than it is a guaranteed right. Abusing the privilege in any way may mean forfeiting your ability to have your pain treated. Thankfully, the responsibilities of pain-management patients are not too difficult to take at this point. But taking the responsibilities as seriously as possible is a must to avoid inconveniences, misunderstandings and more importantly, needless suffering.

Your responsibilities as patient.

1) Arrive at your clinic visits on time. The initial visit will likely require paper work to fill out, unless it had been mailed you previously. The schedules in many pain practices are "tight" and do not allow a lot or room for lateness. Even with the most efficient clinics, unforeseen events occur, which pressurize the schedule even more. Don't contribute to the problem by being late. If legitimate circumstances arise that may

cause you to be late, call ahead and re-schedule if necessary. Also if you are ill with the cold or flu, call ahead to be rescheduled for when you are well.

2) Be courteous and respectful to the provider and staff members. A pain clinic is obviously not the "happiest place on earth", because people are in pain. When people experience pain, they can become angry. It is possible that before you have checked in for your visit, the receptionists, nursing staff and doctor have all experienced the brunt of someone's anger. They pledge to not let that bad experience filter over into your experience with them, so do your best to do the same. Some clinics will dismiss a patient permanently for rude behavior, profanity or belligerence. You probably feel the same way about your job environment.

3) Be courteous and respectful to the other patients in the waiting areas. They are in pain. This is not a time for them to experience additional discomfort or stress. The clinic waiting room is not a day care.

Disruption and noises, particularly from young children, can be aggravating. Make sure that if you have children that you make arrangements for their care, so that the focus can be on you.

Also, be careful not to judge people. Pain can have a devastating impact on a person financially, emotionally, and spiritually. Don't be surprised if there is a person in the waiting room who is not dressed in the best clothes, or is wearing makeup, has the best hygiene, or looks "professional". They may have been nothing like that before they became a victim of pain. You may never know the story behind what led them to the present point. Treat them like you expect to be treated__with respect and dignity.

4) Do not discuss your medications with anyone outside of your treatment providers. It is not wise to do so. This definitely includes strangers in the waiting area, and may extend to your own friends and family, and perhaps, even your spouse. The rationale for this is privacy. You really don't know the person sitting next to you. They may be an undercover agent, wanting to "buy ' your

medicines. They may be someone who follows you to the pharmacy and follows you home to rob you of the medications you just told them you had. This happens.

Also, in some cases, it may not be safe to disclose your medications to your friends and family. They may not understand your pain. They may not approve of your treatment with pain medications. This can cause a significant riff in a family, so whereas they can know you are under a doctors care, they do not necessarily need to know what medications you are prescribed. Similarly, your best friends will probably protect your interest and privacy, but who is to say that your best-friend's 16-year-old son and his friends will do so, if they happens to find out you have pain medications from a doctor in your house. What I have explained to patients is that if you would not tell your friend or neighbor you have 'Herpes' or other sexually-transmissable diseases, then why would you tell them about what pain medications you are on. Exceptions may include your employer, who may have a need to know what medications you take. This is particularly important for people who are truck-drivers, work with patients or operate heavy-equipment. The time for your employer to find out that you take pain medication is not after you take a random drug test at work or after an on-the-job accident. It is before. I would not fear having your employer disclose your health-information. Doing so would be against the law. Friends and Neighbors, on the other hand, are not bound by this. Some also question the recommendations to avoid letting your spouse know about your medications.   This is a personal decision for you to make. Sometimes, spouses on one day, become ex-spouses on another day. And vindictiveness can lead to unfortunate situations which could be avoid if you had not armed them with the information to harm you.

5) Do not be afraid to communicate your pain to your doctor and the assistants. There is no need to under-report or over-exaggerate your pain. It is what it is. Also, be completely honest about how your medication is working. For example, if you report a 10 out-of-10 rating on the pain scale after medication has been given to you, don't be surprised if that medication is taken away. Why would a doctor continue to prescribe a controlled medication that made you no better with it than you were without it? If, on the other, you communicate that the medication is

helping you, but not to the degree that you would like it be, the doctor may be able to make an adjustment to the medication that is acceptable to you.

6) Take your medications as prescribed. Do not overtake your medications under any circumstances. You may discontinue the medication if you are having a reaction to it or cannot tolerate it. If this happens, the doctor should be informed as soon as possible.

7) Do not take any medications for pain other than those that have been prescribed to you by your pain doctor. This means do not ask or do not accept any other medications for pain from any other doctor, or any other person (friend, family, stranger). This is designed as a safety measure that helps prevent you from overdosing or becoming addicted. Exceptions to this rule may occur in true emergencies, dental procedures (with the foreknowledge and approval by your pain doctor, and major surgical procedures requiring medicine above what you are

prescribed for your baseline chronic pain. Also, if your regular provider wants to prescribe a codeine-based medicine for your cough or cold, then, in general, this is permissible so long as your pain-management doctor is aware. He or she may want to prescribe it for you. If not, at least your pain doctor will be able to document this occurrence in your chart should anyone (The pharmacy, or state regulatory agency) question your medication usage. If you experience an emergency after normal clinic hours, please communicate that you are being currently treated for chronic pain with the physician at the emergency room. And at the earliest available moment, inform your pain-management doctor of the situation.

8) Do not give or loan your medications to anyone. Do not sell your medications to anyone. This includes your best friend, sibling, parent, child or neighbor. It does not matter how much pain you think they are in. Not only is this a violation of your agreement with your physician, but this is a violation of law, a felony that could land you in jail. The person you think you can trust may be a

proxy for an undercover law-enforcement agent. Additionally, a medication prescribed for you may not be safe for another person. Explaining that you gave your medication to someone else, who took it and then stopped breathing, is a situation that you do not want to ever face. Also, be prepared to report to your provider and to law-enforcement situations where you were asked to buy or sell medications. Those who participate in this type of criminal activity are ones who have made pain-management less accessible to those like you who are law-abiding.

9) Always keep your medication secure from theft or inadvertent destruction. Because of the "street value" that certain pain medications command, theft of these medications is common. Thefts have even been reported as patients are leaving their pharmacies, or when people leave their purses or briefcases, containing the pill bottles and medication unattended. Once a month's worth of medication has been filled, it cannot be replaced under normal circumstances. So protect your pain medication like you would protect a hundred-dollar bill. Keeping your

medicine in your bathroom cabinet may not be safe as all potential thieves who enter your home, invited or uninvited, know that that location is the first place to look. Some people, particular those who live in a home where other residents have known substance-abuse issue use a safe for their medications. If with all of these precautions, your medications end up stolen, this matter should be reported to law enforcement. Even though, no perpetrator may be charged or punished, you have defense if the pill bottle with your name shows up in a teenagers car after he hits and kills a family of five. You will be thankful that you reported your medications stolen prior to this tragedy.

10)   Be prepared to provide a urine sample at each visit. Urine testing is also becoming a standard part of the assessment of pain-management patients. Dialysis patients or patients with difficulty urinating due to previous surgery or prostate enlargement are exceptions. A note may be required from your urologist documenting the inability or difficulty. In general, the sample you give is analyzed at the clinic while you are there as a quick "qualitative" test for the substances

present in like your medications and the substances (illegal drugs) that should not be present in your sample. The rest of the sample is sent to a reference lab, usually outside of the office, for "quantitative analysis" or confirmation of the amounts of those substances in your urine. This is important, because a specific pain medicine taken 4-times-a-day will show up in the quantitative test differently than a medication that is taken once-a-day. A person who overtakes their medicine and runs out of medicine ahead of schedule will also be identifiable in this testing. Patients who take their medications as prescribed have nothing to fear with these tests. Patients who do not comply, do have a lot to fear from these tests. The provider however is able to document your compliance, and is able to demonstrate to you or anyone else that the pain-management care that you receive is safe. This is not to say testing is fool proof. There are documented false-positives and false-negatives, but typically these occur less that 5% of samples.

11)	Follow the narcotics agreement or contract to the letter. The narcotics contract or agreement is the list of rules and responsibilities, including, but not limited to, the ones above, that you, the patient, agree to prior to the physician agreeing to see you at the beginning of your care. These agreements are becoming standard in most clinics which see pain patients. It may be updated sporadically to reflect changes in office policy or governmental policy.

Chapter 6

What to Do if You are Fired as a Patient

The decision by your provider to terminate the physician-patient relationship is usually not an easy one or one that is taken lightly. In terminating a patient, a doctor loses not only that patient as a client, but his entire network of family or friends that could be referred if they needed pain management. So, the termination is only done when clearly there is no other alternative.

Usually the termination or firing has happened as a result of one the important rules of the narcotic agreement is violated that cannot be overlooked or justified. In actuality, it is not the doctor who terminates you as patient, it is you who terminated the agreement by violating one or more of the rules you have agreed to.

Some terminations are reversible. For example, if you were having a bad day and were in pain, and you let your anger get the best of you momentarily, and in so doing, disrespected the doctor or a staff member. Those types of situations can be salvageable, but it may require an apology and a commitment by you to make sure it never happens again.

Other situations are not negotiable or justifiable. For example, if you sell you medications to a neighbor's teenage son, and the neighbor calls the office to report you, then in most cases you will be terminated immediately, with no hope of reconsideration.   This is true even if the neighbor who calls is just a disgruntled friend who wants to create trouble for you by concocting this story. The reason that most clinics will err on the side of the disgruntled neighbor who may be lying is because of Responsibility #4 from above. How would anyone know who your doctor was and possibly what medications you were taking without them having witness the situation they are reporting? Since you have been advised not discuss your medications with anyone outside of your treatment providers, it can only be presumed that what the caller is reporting is in fact true. The doctor must err on the side of public safety, your safety, and frankly, his or her medical license.

Let's say the doctor or nurse disregarded what the caller reported using the reasoning that since there was no "proof "in a legal sense of the word that what the caller alleges is true. If your doctor decided to prescribe pain medication for you again, and someone was hurt because you actually were selling your medication, your doctor would have to justify why he or she disregarded the information from the caller who essentially handed it to him or her on a silver platter. Because of this type of scenario, you are advised not to disclose your health information regarding your pain-management to anyone outside of your medical care takers, so that there is no possibility of anonymous reporting about abusing your medications. Problem solved.

Another situation which does not leave room for negotiation is a failed urine test. If your urine test shows that there is none of the prescribed medication it, or that the specimen has been tampered with (like bringing urine from the outside source), or the levels are much lower than would be expected based on your dose, then you are not a candidate for continued treatment. If your urine test shows the presence of other pain medications that have not been prescribed to you (e.g., suboxone, methadone or other medication), then this suggests abuse and your termination will be non-negotiable. If your urine tests shows the present of illicit substances like (heroine, cocaine, PCP or Methamphetamine) then it is not safe for you to be prescribed medications for pain and you will be terminated. You should instead be recommended for substance abuse treatment.

If you find yourself in a position where the physician-patient relationship is terminated, and you feel there is a legitimate explanation for the reason you have been given, then I suggest you go home, take some time to think about he situation then write a detailed letter explaining the circumstances clearly. Honesty is your only chance at having the doctor agree to take another chance on you. So, use the opportunity to admit whatever the mistake you made was, and what assurances you can give to make sure that this mistake will never occur again. The chances are very slim to overturn the doctor's decision, the more egregious the violation is, but being open, honest, sincere, contrite and repentant are your best chance for another chance.

Should your written appeal to the doctor fail, then

if you legitimately feel that you have pain that needs to be treated, and you fully understand the shortcomings that lead to your termination from the precious pain doctor, then I suggest you try again with a different doctor. When you are evaluated by the next doctor, make sure you fully disclose the termination by the previous doctor and what will be different if this doctor agrees to take care of you. Most doctors will be impressed with the character you are showing by disclosing this. Some will not. This may be the price you have to pay for a mistake, as we all must do in life. Failure to disclose this in the beginning, however, will only hurt you down the line. Odds are your new doctor will eventually discover the truth. Breaking the bond of trust is hard to forgive an overcome in the pain-management business.

Chapter 7

Pain-Management Resources

You can find a lot of supportive information online from these sources:

Patient Resources

Books

Your Aching Back: A Doctors Guide to Relief Augustus A White, III MD PhD, with Prestion J. Phillips MD

Heal Your Aching Back: What A Harvard Doctor Wants you to Know About Finding Relief & Keeping your Back Strong

On the Web

GivingPainAVoice In Oklahoma/#338Strong

www.GivingPainAVoiceInOklahoma.com

American Chronic Pain Association

www.theapca.org

Power of Pain National Pain Foundation

www.powerofpain.org

PainEDU

www.painedu.org

Partners Against Pain

www.partnersagainstpain.com

National Fibromyalgia & Chronic Pain Association

www.fmcpaware.org

The Pain Community

www.paincommunity.org

For Clinicians

American Pain Society

www.americanpainsociety.org

American Academy of Pain Medicine

www.painmed.org

American Academy of Pain Management

www.aapainmanage.org

Pain Policy/Advocacy

Pain & Policy Studies Group

www.painpolicy.wisc.edu

Drug Policy Alliance

www.drugpolicy.org

Blogs

Back and Neck Pain Blog

www.spine-health.com/blog

Institute for Chronic Pain Blog

www.instituteforchronicpain.org/blog/

All Flared Up RA Blog

www.allflaredup.wordpress.com

Fibro & Fabulous/ Fibromyalgia Blog

www.fibroandfabulous.com

Other Books by this Author …

Please check out the next book in my Pain-Management series called:

"5 Ways to Effortlessly Outsmart Your Pain Doctor"

available on Amazon Kindle

http://amzn.to/1b3sBhb

Below are some of my future titles, which if you liked this book, I am confident you will enjoy as well, maybe even more.

Be on the look out for:

"The Cheat Sheet"

and

"Dealer (Fiction)"

Coming Soon!

One Last Thing...

When you turn the page, Kindle will give you the opportunity to rate the book and share your thoughts on Facebook and Twitter. If you believe the book is worth sharing, would you take a few seconds to let your friends know about it? If it turns out to make a difference in their lives, they'll be forever grateful to you. As will I.

All my best,
Harvey Jenkins, MD PhD

www.ingramcontent.com/pod-product-compliance
Lightning Source LLC
Chambersburg PA
CBHW041311210326
41599CB00003B/66